"But You LOOK Good"

How to Encourage and Understand People Living with Illness and Pain

Wayne and Sherri Connell

Invisible Disabilities Association
www.InvisibleDisabilities.org

Published by the Invisible Disabilities® Association

First Printing 1998
Reprinted 1998 – 2014
Over 28,000 Copies in Print

For ordering information or special discounts for bulk purchases, contact IDA P.O. Box 4067 Parker, CO 80134, orders@invisibledisabilities.org

Written by Wayne and Sherri Connell
Edited by Carole Mitchell and Kris Harty
Cover Design by Wes Connell

ISBN 978-0-692-25845-3

But You LOOK Good is not intended as professional advice. It is solely informational. Please seek the advice of a professional.

All proceeds support the Invisible Disabilities® Association, a 501(c)(3) Non-Profit whose mission is to encourage, educate and connect people and organizations touched by illness, pain and disability around the globe.

Invisible Disabilities Association
P.O. Box 4067
Parker, Colorado 80134
Website: www.InvisibleDisabilities.org

Contents

Invisible Disabilities Association

Founder and President, Wayne Connell, saw the need to establish the *Invisible Disabilities® Association,* originally known as *The Invisible Disabilities Advocate®,* as a place of compassion and understanding for those living with debilitating illness, pain and injury. Wayne's inspiration to create this organization came from his wife, Sherri, who became disabled at the age of 27. He is joined by business, medical and scientific professionals to reach out to the world with IDA's message.

Often the most difficult part of living with a debilitating illness or injury is the lack of understanding the person encounters. Since most living with a chronic condition do not always look sick to us, we find ourselves struggling to believe their limitations are real. Even when our friend or family member tells us they are unable to work, attend a gathering, shop, cook, clean, etc., we often disregard what they are *saying,* because we think they look fine!

Let's face it; most people cannot comprehend what it is like to be sick or in pain for weeks, months or even years, because we are used to going to the doctor, taking some medication and soon feeling better. Consequently, unless we are educated about what life changes a chronic condition can bring, we may inadvertently treat our loved one as if they just need to "snap out of it" or "stop complaining." As a result, the only way to transform our well-meaning, but hurtful view is to understand that the illness can debilitate a person's body - *against the person's will!*

Therefore, the Invisible Disabilities® Association strives to explain that even though the symptoms from chronic illness, pain and injury may not always be obvious to us, these invisible disabilities are real. IDA provides helpful links to sites and organizations of several diseases, disorders and conditions, as well as a support board.

Most of all, IDA offers informative articles and this book, *But You LOOK Good, which* can be handed out to friends, family, support groups and co-workers, to help them to understand the challenges and difficulties of living with a disease or injury that can be debilitating.

But You LOOK Good serves as a guide to understanding, encouraging and helping those who are limited by their condition. Even more, IDA helps people see the courage and strength their loved one has displayed, despite their losses, limitations and daily challenges.

Let us not treat those who are ill or have been injured as if they are lazy or malingering. Instead, let us take a closer look at what courage and strength it takes to live with a physical limitation. After all, they are displaying perseverance through personal loss and endurance despite disappointment that most people fortunately will never know.

What is an Invisible Disability?

"A person is considered to have a disability if he or she has difficulty performing certain functions (seeing, hearing, talking, walking, climbing stairs and lifting and carrying), or has difficulty performing activities of daily living, or has difficulty with certain social roles (doing school work for children, working at a job and around the house for adults)."[1] Just because a person has a disability, does not mean they are "disabled." Many living with physical or mental challenges are still able to be active in their hobbies, work and sports. On the other hand, some struggle to get through their day at work and some cannot work at all.

Often, when we think of the term, "disability," we assume it only refers to people using a wheelchair or walker. On the contrary, the 1994-1995 Survey of Income and Program Participation (SIPP) found that 26 million Americans (almost 1 in 10) were considered to have a severe disability, while only 1.8 million used a wheelchair and 5.2 million used a cane, crutches or walker.[2] In other words, 74% of Americans who live with a severe disability do not use such devices. In view of that, a disability cannot be determined solely on whether or not a person uses assistive equipment.

The term *invisible disability* refers to a person's symptoms, such as extreme fatigue, dizziness, pain, weakness, cognitive impairments, etc. that are sometimes or always debilitating. These symptoms can occur due to chronic illness, chronic pain, injury, birth disorders, etc. and are not always obvious to the onlooker.

A person can have an invisible disability whether or not they have a visible impairment or use an assistive device like a wheelchair, walker, cane, etc. For example, a person utilizing a wheelchair may be restricted by their pain, fatigue and/or cognitive dysfunctions. Accordingly, these symptoms are their invisible disabilities.

About the Book

"But You LOOK Good" gives those living with chronic illness and pain a voice about how they feel, what they need and how others can be an encouragement to them. It is a convenient, informative way to educate loved ones about what people living with ongoing illness and pain struggle with, fight for and need from their friends and family. It is easy to read, gives practical ideas on how loved ones can be supportive and is in an ideal, condensed length for busy readers.

This booklet gets to the heart of why our friends and family have difficulty with understanding ongoing illness and pain. It serves as a tool to help explain to loved ones how extreme symptoms (fatigue, pain, dizziness, cognitive impairments and other symptoms) can be limiting, although the person may not look sick or in pain. Moreover, it gives them simple, pragmatic ways to truly be an encouragement: *What to say*, *What not to say and Why*, along with *How to help*. Often, loved ones are enlightened by this book as to why their well-meaning advice is not always well-received. It is cherished by both those living with illness or injury, as well as those who love them!

"But You LOOK Good" is printed and distributed by the Invisible Disabilities Association. It is based upon the knowledge learned by the life experiences of Wayne and Sherri Connell, as well as countless others who live with debilitating conditions.

About the Authors

All of her life, Sherri Connell was an extremely active person who loved her careers, singing and dancing in musicals, modeling, riding her horse and lifting weights. She started having health problems when she was 14, but did not know why. Despite chronic headaches, constant bouts with strep throat, the flu and bronchial pneumonia, Sherri was an active, goal-oriented "go-getter." In college, she studied Music Theatre, and then obtained two Bachelor's degrees in Business, with a Minor in Liberal Arts.

Although Sherri had enormous plans and goals, her life took an unexpected turn. As she was plotting out her Master's degree, she was stopped in her tracks at the age of 27. Starting with another winter bout of pneumonia, Sherri became paralyzed and so sick she could barely sit up. She was hospitalized and diagnosed with Progressive Multiple Sclerosis. It was later discovered she also had Late-Chronic Lyme Disease from a tick bite when she was 14. The diagnosis did not scare her, because she figured she could still work and sing from a wheelchair. Nothing had ever stopped her before and nothing was going to stop her now!

Much to her dismay, her health never improved, but quickly worsened. Due to extreme flu-like symptoms such as bone-crushing fatigue, severe nerve pain, cognitive dysfunctions, memory loss, dizziness, heart arrhythmias, weakness, nausea and migraines, Sherri was never able to return to work. This was extremely difficult for her, because she had been working since she was 13 and her work was her life! She did regain some of the use of her legs through much rehabilitation, but she still cannot stand long or walk far. Sherri's life suddenly went from "on the go 24/7" to struggling to get to a doctor's appointment, prepare a meal or take a shower.

Despite the seriousness of Sherri's illness, people often had difficulty understanding how she could look good and be as sick as she was. Unfortunately, because of these misconceptions, people often jumped to the conclusion that she was lazy, unmotivated or not trying hard enough. For a goal-oriented, talented, career-driven person like Sherri, these notions were absolutely devastating. In fact, Sherri wanted her life back more than anything. She continued to go from doctor to doctor, as well as try countless treatments, therapies and surgeries.

Unfortunately, Sherri remained plagued by hurtful comments and assumptions from those around her. Determined to grasp how people came to these conclusions, she began writing in her journal about her losses and the responses of others. "The process of forming thoughts into words and the physical act of drawing the hand across the page... slows rushing thoughts and pulls the attention into focus."[3] Since Sherri continued to grapple with verbally explaining to people what she was going through, she began printing copies from her journal to share with others.

One day her husband, Wayne Connell, offered to post some of her writing on the internet so that they could tell people, "Go check out the Web site," instead of stumbling to find the words to explain. Much to Wayne and Sherri's amazement, as the word spread like wildfire across the internet, emails started pouring in from people around the globe. These readers who lived with various chronic conditions told countless personal stories of losing cherished relationships with friends and family members, because of the complexities of their invisible disabilities. Nonetheless, people were ecstatic to tell Wayne and Sherri that the articles had put into words exactly what they had been trying to say to their loved ones.

Wayne then discovered there were millions of other people around the world being hurt by the same lack of understanding and belief that Sherri was experiencing. His passion quickly grew from being his wife's supporter, to being an advocate for all who are living with disabilities. In order to create a format that was easy for people to share with their friends and family, Wayne and IDA compiled this booklet, "But You LOOK Good" It serves as a guide, as it contains excerpts from Sherri's journal enlightening people with what to say, what not to say and how to help someone living with a debilitating condition. IDA prints and distributes this booklet to people living with chronic illness and pain, as well as their loved ones. All proceeds go to IDA, a non-profit organization.

Dedication

We would like to dedicate this book to all of you who live with limitations due to chronic illness and pain. We hope you will find comfort, camaraderie and support in this organization. Most of all, we pray your loved ones will develop a better understanding of your loss and battles. May their hearts be softened and their eyes be opened with compassion, respect and belief in you as an *important* and viable human being!

Thanks
From Sherri Connell

First, I would like to thank my family for loving me and standing by my side from the very beginning! I thank you for realizing I never wanted to live with this and have fought it every step of the way! Thank you for respecting me, for believing my word and for seeing me as strong instead of weak! Thank you for treating me like I am just as valuable as I was before and for knowing I would never willingly give up my dreams, aspirations and lifelong goals! Finally, I would especially like to give credit to the "Greatest Mom in the World," my mom! Thank you! I love you all!

Next, I would like to thank my husband, Wayne, for seeing my perseverance, positive attitude and courage when we met. I thank you for looking *beyond* my limitations and for treating me as a whole person, just as valuable as I was when I had a career or could sing and dance on stage. You did not know me back then, but you loved me for the person I was inside and not for what I did for a living. Incredibly, you stand beside me when friends, loved ones and strangers continue to make comments that cause deep, deep pain. When it seems like everyone else is treating me like I am *choosing* this illness, your faith in me *never* ceases! You are my protector and my best friend.

Wayne, I also want to thank you for providing a platform for reaching out to others debilitated by illness and pain. You have done so much to share what I have gone through with others who are also struggling with so many losses and misunderstanding among loved ones. Thank you for doing what I never could have done myself!

Most of all, I want to thank God for loving me and for helping me to live with this painful disability. Though I am weak, you are my strength to go on. I do not know why you have not healed my body, but I do know you have promised the healing of my soul and a new body when I am joined with you forever. I thank you for preparing for me a place in heaven and giving me hope of eternal life in your presence!

Special Thanks

We want to say a special thank you to a few of the people who have helped financially to make the printing of this book possible; Kim Blackerby, Rick Fort, Steve Hardardt, Lloyd Lewis and John Kelley.

Foreword
A Tribute to an American Heroine

Sometimes a person's character is not evident until thrown into the furnace of affliction; like John Wayne's tough determination wasn't evident in a movie until he was out-gunned ten to one. That is part of what makes Sherri Connell's story so compelling. Against all odds, she emerges as a determined woman of real grit, capable of taking on the meanest that life has to throw at her, and still surfacing with heroic courage after getting hit by a Tsunami. She has always been a person who, as far as I can tell from reading her story, if she died on Tuesday, would probably have shown up to work on Wednesday saying, "I'm not going to let some minor problems like death and a coffin keep me down."

Yet, despite her cussed determination to cling onto the vestiges of "normal life" after a tidal wave of devastation to every system of her body, still her so-called "friends" thought she must be a sissy, giving-in to feelings of being tired, and using illness as an excuse to retreat. Some friends!

Sherri has helped me put into words something that has been knocking around inside my skull as a half-baked idea, namely that some parts of the popular American culture are intensely hostile to those who suffer from chronic illnesses, especially invisible disabilities. That, of course, is not what we Americans think about ourselves. After all, we have given disabled people preferential parking spaces and passed the Americans with Disabilities Act.

But think about it. If you turn on TV or open most popular

magazines, you are confronted with healthy and beautiful bodies of models under the age of thirty. That is what life is supposed to be about, or so we are told. We are all supposed to enjoy our bodies, exercise aerobically, be sexy, and drive glamorous new cars, and remain under the age of thirty without showing any effects of age, gravity or disease. Or at least that is the hype.

We tend to take health, family, food, and other blessings as being our birthright. The thought does not come easily that these are blessings that we don't deserve, that God is free to either give or withhold. The blessings of this life are only a brief and dilute taste of heaven. If Sherri's friends had realized that the purpose of life is to glorify God rather than to enjoy their "birthright" health, then they would have recognized that Sherri was fulfilling that purpose more successfully than they were. If Sherri's friends had understood these points, they would have become more humble.

In a classic article in the Journal of the American Medical Association on November 13, 1996, Catherine Hoffman and Dorothy Rice made an appraisal of the extent and cost of chronic illness in the United States. About 46% of Americans suffer with one chronic condition or another, most of them are employed, most of them are under the age of 65. The cost is staggering, and is the leading cause of the ongoing inflation in the cost of healthcare and prescription drugs.

The fundamental issue is that contemporary medicine is often able to delay death but not restore health, so that the more breakthroughs of modern medicine we have, the more sick people we have. I say this without sarcasm and without cynicism. A century ago, someone like Sherri Connell would have died years ago. She does not think it is bad to be alive, even though she remains crushed by afflictions. God's blessings are still delicious, even when there are fewer of them available to Sherri today than when she was a healthy teenager.

Here's another example of how the miraculous breakthroughs of modern medicine increase the number of sick people. In the old days, if you had a severe head injury, you died of brain swelling. Starting a couple of decades ago, doctors learned how to prevent brain swelling, so that acute brain damage did not necessarily lead to death. But as a result of that breakthrough of medicine, there is a large and rapidly growing number of Americans with Traumatic Brain Injury, most of whom are unable to return to the kind of work and lifestyle they had before, and many of whom are permanently disabled. Thus the more successful medicine is, the more sick people we have among us.

I am beginning to suspect that popular American culture is built upon the pipe-dream that disease has been conquered by physicians, or will soon be conquered as soon as we figure out what all that DNA says. I've been a physician now for a quarter century, and let me assure you that is not how it looks from down here in the trenches. If this were a football game the score would be DISEASE 85 versus DOCTORS 15. Our score of 15 is much higher than it was a century ago. But we are far from winning the game. We lack the power to cure someone like Sherri, alas.

My point is that Sherri Connell's heroic effort to alert her friends to the realities of invisible disabilities is a message that Americans desperately need to hear. Those who believe the TV hype about how the meaning of life requires that you must first possess a healthy and sexy young body, will be humbled as they grow older. The elderly know what it means to live with illness and disability, which sometimes is less severe, and sometimes more, but is always apparent even in the loss of elasticity and thickness from the skin, the growing wrinkles and tendency to droop with the impact of gravity over many decades.

Foreword Written by Jeffrey H. Boyd, M.D., M.Div., M.P.H.
Dr. Boyd is a psychiatrist and Chairman of Waterbury Hospital's Behavioral Health Department in Connecticut. He is also the author of Being Sick Well: Joyful Living Despite Chronic Illness. Dr. Boyd writes and lectures on coping with chronic illness.

Chapter One

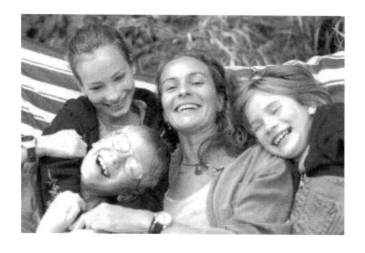

But They LOOK Good!

Do I love you because you're beautiful,
Or are you beautiful because I love you?

~ Cinderella - Rodgers and Hammerstein

What is a Chronic Condition?

A chronic condition is a disease, disorder, birth defect or injury that a person has to cope with on a continuous basis. It also "...lasts a year or longer, limits activity, and may require ongoing care."[4] "As of 2012, about half of all adults—117 million people—have one or more chronic health conditions. One of four adults has two or more chronic health conditions."[5]

Sometimes an illness goes undiagnosed for a very long time, leaving people frustrated, discouraged and without answers to why their bodies will not cooperate with their desires. When they do get a diagnosis, it often takes months or sometimes years to regulate the medications. Many continue to adjust their prescriptions and vie with side effects for an ongoing basis. Some try dozens of therapies, prescriptions, treatments and procedures, remaining unable to function to some degree.

People living with chronic conditions often vary in severity. Many have mild symptoms, and with a little adjustment in their diets or schedules, they can lead a normal life. Some have to make bigger changes by avoiding various activities or cutting back their work. Others are unable to work at all and struggle to get through life's daily needs.

But They Don't "LOOK" Sick!

As previously stated, 74% of Americans considered to have a severe disability do not use a wheelchair, walker, cane or crutches. Therefore, we should not always expect a disability obvious to the onlooker. Moreover, whether or not a person uses an assistive device, their symptoms such as extreme fatigue, pain, dizziness, cognitive impairments, blurred vision, etc. can be mild to severely debilitating.

The truth is "Many with chronic physical illness look no different than other people..."[6] revealed Pauline Boss, PhD, a professor of Family Social Science at The University of Minnesota. For example, most neurological, immunological, genetic, organ, brain, blood and skeletal disorders due to disease, dysfunctions, birth defects and injuries and are not readily apparent to others. Even so, they may be keeping the person from being as active as they once were.

Because of this, families and friends often struggle with understanding how their loved one can look fine, but say they are ill or in pain. Lynn, a woman with Multiple Sclerosis expressed, "I have gone from being super-mom, PTA president, volunteer of the year, super organized to barely being able to get out of bed in the morning on some days. I feel like no one understands why I'm not able to do the same things anymore...because *I look fine!* I can't remember a lot of things now, can't run on the treadmill, have to sit and rest 20 times a day...but *I look fine! I must just be lazy!"*[7]

Clearly, we must not expect to see a disease that lives below the skin, because most illnesses are not obvious from the outside. After all, doctors usually require x-rays, MRIs, microscopes and blood tests, etc. to diagnose a disease or disorder, because we cannot see most illnesses from the outside. As a result, instead of questioning our loved one's complaints, we simply need to believe what they are saying is true - *even if we cannot see it.*

They Have Good and Bad Days, Right?

Actually, not everyone with a chronic condition has the same symptoms or degree of symptoms. People with the same diagnosis can have varying limitations and severity. In general, there are basically three stages in a chronic illness:

THE EARLY STAGE: This person may notice occasional symptoms or lack of energy. Once in a while, they experience setbacks from a few activities. If diagnosed in this stage, many can get help from their doctors and utilize proper nutrition to prevent further progression of the disease and still lead a very active life. *This person has mostly good days with occasional bad days.*

THE MIDDLE STAGE (or the Relapsing/Remitting Stage): This person may experience occasional to frequent bouts with symptoms. They must learn not to overexert themselves in order to avoid relapse of illness and increased symptoms. Many can lower the frequency of relapse and progression of the disease with help from their doctors and proper nutrition. *This person has both good and bad days, depending on activity, stress and treatment.*

THE LATE STAGE (or the Progressive Stage): This person's disease has progressed to the point where it usually does not remit. They may regularly live with symptoms that feel much like having the flu, complete with extreme fatigue, muscle aches, weakness, pain, nausea, cognitive difficulties, dizziness, etc. People in this stage may not respond as well to treatment. *This person may have very few good days.*

In all, for those living with both good and bad days, it is fine for us to ask them how they are feeling or if they are having a good day. Then, we can rejoice with them for the days they are doing well. However, for those who feel bad every day, it is not necessary for us to ask them how they are *feeling* all of the time. Instead, we can ask them how they are *doing*. This allows the person to answer regarding their outlook on life, despite their hurdles.

What's more, because we see someone out and about, does not mean it is because they are having a good day. As a matter of fact, many living with chronic illness cannot wait for a good day in order to buy groceries or run an errand. So, we should not assume they are doing well, but instead realize that they are probably going to be feeling worse from the endeavor.

For many living with an illness or disorder, their lives are greatly affected until they are able to improve with various therapies. On the other hand, for others it is an ongoing endeavor to find something that will allow them to get part or all of their lives back.

This booklet will mainly address those who regularly experience being debilitated by an illness or injury, even though they have made great efforts to get better. We will discuss the struggle of having limitations during a relapse, whether it lasts for several days, weeks or even years at a time. We suggest our readers ask their loved one for information on their particular diagnosis, as well as about their individual symptoms and frequency of symptoms. This will help you to have a better understanding of the level of challenges they might be facing.

I Just Don't Understand!

At least once in our lives, most of us have experienced having to stay home from work or school because we were too sick to go. Here, we are not talking about a day where we might have felt a little under the weather, so we decided to call in sick in order to catch up on our laundry or our errands!

No, we are referring to the day where just sitting up or talking took great effort and a fever made every muscle ache, right down to the bone. Remember how hard trying to get up to go to the bathroom was? Your head would pound, your body felt like it weighed a ton and you became dizzy and nauseous.

You may even remember having been hurt in an accident and forced to give up activities you loved for a few weeks or even a few months. Thus, you know how stressful and depressing it can be when you are unable to do what you want to do.

We have yet to meet someone who is really down with a cold, flu or injury tell us they are having the time of their lives and enjoying every minute of it. On the contrary, most people become frustrated and impatient after just a few hours of being sick. If it lasts more than a day or two, we quickly panic about missing work, school or other activities and we groan about the discomfort.

The irony is that even though we cannot stand to miss a few days out of *our* lives, we still often treat our loved ones with ongoing conditions as if losing long periods of *their* lives should not be any big deal. Instead of showing them compassion for their losses and frustrations, we often try to tell them it is not that bad. Nevertheless, if we can recognize our own feelings about being sick or in pain, we can certainly understand that it is no fun for our loved one either, and we can learn to show compassion.

It is true that most people can never fully comprehend what it is like to live with an illness or pain on an ongoing basis. Most will never completely grasp the loss of activities, independence and careers. Lyme Disease patient, Geri Fosseen exclaimed, "Welcome to the world of invisible chronic illness. This is a hard world to live in, one in which you're positive no one could possibly understand how hard it is to live like this."[8]

We may never totally understand, yet we can still have an understanding. We like to give the analogy of an airplane. We may not fully understand how it flies, but we have an understanding or belief that it does. Just the same, we may not completely understand how our loved one feels or why, but we can have an understanding or belief that they do. In light of that, let us stop focusing on what we do not understand and start focusing on simply believing what our loved one says is true.

Because all of us know how difficult it is to be sick or injured and forced to put our lives on hold for a while, we know we would not want to feel this way ourselves. Our loved one wants us to see their courage as they endure this marathon before them. Consequently, let us tell them how amazed we are at their strength and perseverance.

What If They Give In to the Illness?

When a promising athlete is injured and faces the possibility of losing all of which he or she has worked so hard to achieve, we cringe when we hear the news. The mere thought of them losing their hopes and dreams makes us realize how devastating it would be for them. Yet, when a loved one loses their job or is forced to give up various activities due to illness, we can be oblivious to the fact that they have lost all for which they have worked, planned and hoped for their future. Sadly, we sometimes assume they have a choice in the matter and are choosing to give in to the illness.

Founder of Rest Ministries, Lisa Copen shared, "When we have a chronic illness, it can be a difficult thing for a friend to understand our changing lifestyle. Perhaps you aren't able to participate in the activities you once did together. Maybe she thinks if you just tried a little harder you could beat the illness. 'You've got to fight this!' is something I've heard on more than one occasion. Despite these friends' good intentions, it puts me on the defensive, trying to prove that I am fighting in the best way I know how."[9]

Therefore, if we believe that our loved one is giving in to the illness, most likely, this is just our perception of how they are handling new limitations. When a person first experiences the effects of a chronic illness, it is common to have a fantastic attitude about conquering it. They feel strong and invincible against its grip. As the disease progresses and they show signs of frustration, they may continue to crusade for their right to live the way they planned their lives to be. What is more, they will stay persistent in the battle until their bodies force them to make limitations.

After all, no one wants to be sick and no one ever chooses to give up those things in life that bring such joy. However, when a condition is ongoing, worsening or exacerbated by overexertion, the person must develop boundaries in order to better manage their situation. Creating limitations for oneself is one of the hardest things a person can do and it goes against everything we are and everything we ever hoped to be. Notwithstanding, these limitations are mandatory in managing a chronic illness. As a result, we must respect these new boundaries by supporting our loved one's need to say, "No," whether or not we understand why.

Learn To See With Your Ears

Chapter Two

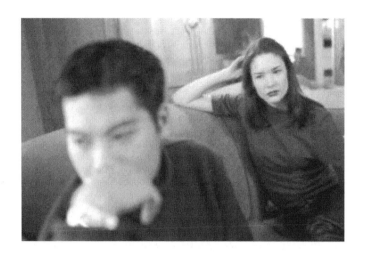

I Can Never Get it Right!

It is the greatest of all mistakes

to do nothing

because you can only do little

- do what you can.

~ Sydney Smith

Why Can't I Say the Right Thing?

Have you ever wanted to encourage your friend or family member, but it seems like you never know what to say? Furthermore, when you finally think of something you know will make them smile, are you shocked when they just snap back at you with frustration? Actually, you are not alone, because "To a healthy person, none of these comments seem unusual or insincere. [We] are simply trying to find the right thing to say."[10] In spite of this, we are often left feeling as if we can never say anything right.

When someone lives with a chronic condition that becomes debilitating, the changes can be very difficult. Obviously, no one can fully understand the depths of the consequences of ongoing illness and pain unless they have experienced them firsthand. Yet, our loved one needs us to at least believe their word is true.

The greatest error we can make is to only believe what they are saying if we can see it. When we disbelieve what they are saying, because we cannot see it, we are attacking their integrity. On the contrary, trusting and believing our friend or family member is not only possible, but it is crucial and absolutely vital. "The importance of conveying respect and integrity while delivering hope cannot be overemphasized…"[11] stressed F. Marcus Brown III, PhD, a therapist who specializes in coping with chronic illness.

The tearing apart of relationships can oftentimes be harder to bear than the illness itself. "If a person is stricken with a disease, his or her level of distress will vary enormously depending on whether the person is isolated (no friends) or has a social network."[12] In order to preserve the relationship, we must believe our loved one and acknowledge the situation at hand to create an environment of support. By listening to their feelings about losses and concerns, we offer them the foundation they need to combat the illness. We can also encourage our loved one by showing them they are still as valuable to us as they were before. These actions will allow them to use their energy to persevere in the race, rather than using it to vie for our belief and trust.

Those who live with chronic conditions want to laugh, smile, look their best and enjoy life. After all, it is their incredible courage, determination and persistence to fight for their lives, which make their illnesses and injuries seem invisible to the naked eye.

The intent of this booklet is to list some *dos* and *don'ts* and to explain how some well-meaning comments can be painful to someone with an illness or injury. You may not understand it completely, because you are not the one battling a disease or injury. Nonetheless, if you desire to encourage your loved one, rather than to discourage them... read on.

Can't I Try to Cheer Them Up?

We must remember that to our loved one, we are only communicating a lack of compassion and sensitivity when we say things like "buck up and live with it" or "just be positive." Even more, what we must learn is that most likely they *do* have a positive attitude.

After all, most people get frustrated with being sick or in pain after a few days or a few hours. For someone living with a persistent illness or injury, it takes an incredibly positive attitude to keep persevering. Think of what a great outlook it must take to contend with limiting symptoms that last for months or even years.

Subsequently, we must not expect them to always be happy about their circumstances. They will smile when we are compassionate about what they are going through, not when we tell them it is not that bad. What's more, they will have a much better attitude when they do not have to grasp for our support.

We realize most people honestly mean well and want to fix the problem, because it is so difficult to watch a loved one suffer. Therefore, we really do understand the desire to make it all better with advice and well-meaning comments. However, the purpose of this booklet is to explain why some of the answers we have may be hurtful and actually make us seem as if we really do not care at all.

If, after reading this booklet, you find that you are unable to communicate positively when talking to your loved one about his or her condition, you might stick with conversation that does not address the illness at all. For those living with debilitating illness and pain, it is much easier to be around people who do not discuss the illness in any way, rather than people who give pat answers, advice and make hurtful comments. Living with a chronic condition and its limitations is difficult enough in and of itself. Our loved one does not need to feel as if they are striving for our belief, respect and compassion, on top of fighting their illness.

Why Do I Respond This Way?

Commonly, those who love someone living with an ongoing

illness or injury tend to remain stuck in the stage of denial. We do this in attempt to protect ourselves and our loved one. Be that as it may, this can be quite difficult, frustrating and hurtful. When we remain in this stage, action, love and practical problem solving does not take place. Columnist Karen J. Zielinski, who has lived with Multiple Sclerosis for over 25 years, wrote, "Denial can be a real devil for people with MS, their friends, family members and their employers."[13]

It is perfectly normal to enter into denial in the beginning, but we often fail to move to the next step of acceptance. We often think that accepting means giving in and allowing the disorder to win. On the contrary, what it really means is to acknowledge that the hurdles are there, so we can execute a plan on how to get over them. This is a very crucial step, because if we ignore it, we will be unable to devise a strategy to cope and endure.

Along with denial, there are four basic, natural reactions that occur in response to seeing a loved one become ill. Although these reactions are normal, they are often followed by comments which make it apparent to our loved one that we are refusing to stand alongside to support him or her in what they have lost and what they are facing.

1) We truly do care and do not want them to have to go through this ordeal. Therefore, we want to fix it by giving advice. However, our suggestions are often impractical or inapplicable. These comments may leave our loved ones thinking we believe they are not trying to get better.

2) We cannot bear to see them suffer so deeply. Therefore, we try to minimize the severity of the situation by continually telling them "It is not so bad" or "It could be worse," etc. However, these comments show we are unwilling to really delve into reality and be compassionate.

3) We fear acknowledging the reality of a disease means giving in to the disease. Therefore, we combat our loved one's statements of fact about their illness. However, by persistently refusing to listen to the information and arguing with their diagnosis, we are refusing to stand by them in order to help them deal with the illness at hand. Notably, we cannot begin to contend with the illness until we know and accept the facts.

4) We need desperately to believe we are in complete control of our own health. We want to believe that we have the answers, so if it happened to us we would be able to avoid the consequences. Therefore, we often find fault in what our friend or family member is doing, so we can continue to believe that illness and pain could be evaded. However, it is destructive to treat our loved one this way. They did not ask for this condition and they are trying everything possible to gain control of it, as well.

As a whole, our reactions are perfectly normal. Nevertheless, when we continue to act as if our loved one's losses are not a big deal, tell them they have to be fixed and treat them as if they are at fault, those faced with a continuing condition will be left feeling alone and isolated in their battle.

It is time for us to move away from denial, and toward acceptance of the facts and acknowledgement of our friend or family member's situation. It will then be apparent that we truly care and that will allow us to be a true source of support. When we give this type of reinforcement, they will not want to quit. Instead, they will want to fight even harder.

Truly Love Me By Believing In Me!

Chapter Three

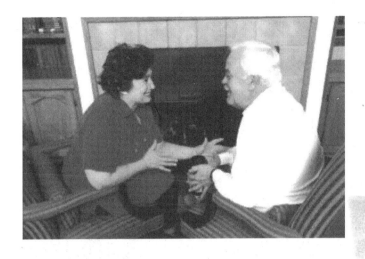

I Never Know What to Say!

Anxiety weighs down the human heart,

but a good word cheers it up.

~ Proverbs 12:25

What Discourages Them?

Most friends and family members truly desire to encourage their loved one. We really do care, are heartbroken over their situation and yearn to help them through it. All the same, many times we may find that our well-meaning comments are not so well-received.

This chapter will give examples of what comments are discouraging, what comments are encouraging and why people living with these conditions feel this way. The following is a list of guidelines to follow, what not to say and why.

Do Not Claim It Doesn't Exist Because You Cannot See It

"But you look good!" "But you don't look sick!"
"It's all in your head." "You just want attention."

When most people are sick with the flu or a fever, they become pale and droopy and their hair is in a tussle. Because of this, when we meet someone who tells us they are ill, but they do not look sick, we are often perplexed. Even so, we must realize that there is a difference between having a cold or the flu and having a chronic illness.

Again, most chronic conditions are not always as perceptible as a bad case of the flu. For instance, a person can battle such symptoms as extreme fatigue or cognitive impairments on the inside, even though they may appear healthy and well on the outside. Just the same, a person can have horrible pain or dizziness, despite the fact that they may seem strong and able.

The biggest grievance those living with chronic conditions have is when people tell them, *"But you look good."* You might be surprised to learn this does not mean they do not want to look good. In fact, people living with chronic illness and pain want to look their best and would welcome a compliment. Nevertheless, when this phrase is used to convey disbelief that the person's condition is real, it is not used as a compliment, but as a dispute.

Here is an example: A scenario that often plays out is when our loved one tells us about their illness or injury. Instead of listening and acknowledging what they are telling us, we refute what they are saying by declaring, *"But you look good."* Regrettably, when we reply this way, our loved one will often hear, *"I don't believe you, because I can't see it for myself."* Evidently, "Peoples' observations do not conform to their expectation as to what a sick person should look and act like. Therefore they are quick to become intolerant and suspect that the symptoms are overstated."[14]

Kristine, a woman living with a difficult disorder wrote, "I just want people to understand that even if we look ok we are still sick. I just had brain surgery and because they didn't shave me bald people look at me like I'm nuts. My family won't accept the fact of my illness that I have had for almost 9 years."[15]

Unfortunately, great strains are forced onto relationships when friends, family and strangers doubt a condition really exists or is truly as limiting as they claim. Sadly, this can be devastating for our friend or family member to hear that others do not believe what they are saying. It makes them feel as if the rug is being pulled out from under them, as we stand in disbelief of their word.

Geri Fosseen, Lyme Disease patient and director of the Ames Chapter of the Iowa Lyme Disease Foundation, dedicated her life to helping people understand debilitating illness, until she died at the age of 31. Fosseen wrote, "'Oh, but you look good!' they say, thinking they're making you feel better. Inside, your stomach grows tight, you inwardly cringe, and fight the urge to scream. 'Oh No! Not this again!' you think!"[16]

Overall, we must resist the temptation to make a visual diagnosis by coming to the conclusion that our loved one must be embellishing their situation or trying to pull the wool over our eyes, because to us they look fine.

Do Not Minimize Their Situation

"It is not that bad!" "It could be worse!"
"You're lucky you don't have to work!"

Often when we come across someone living with a debilitating condition, we question if it is really as bad as they claim. This is not unusual, because people with such perplexing conditions, "...often face doctors who don't take their symptoms seriously, as well as friends and co-workers who think they're over-dramatizing their problems."[17]

Telling our loved one "It is not that bad" can be hurtful, because we are acting as if having hopes, dreams and desires limited by a disorder is no big deal. Unless we are in our loved one's shoes, we should not tell them "It could be worse."

True, there are often people worse off and it is always good to remember to be thankful for what we do have. Then again, even though there is probably someone worse off, that does not make all our loved one's losses go away. When we say this, it seems as if we are discounting what they have lost and are facing. This is a comment that should be reserved for the person living with the limiting condition to say.

The bottom line is people living with debilitating disorders experience varying degrees of limitations from no longer being able to do it all, to barely struggling to do anything. It can be overwhelming when the losses pile up, so they will need to be addressed. After all, "A chronically ill person is likely to endure multiple losses that may include the loss of control and personal power, which is an important contributor to self- esteem, as well as loss of independence, loss of identity, loss of financial status and loss of one's customary lifestyle."[18]

One of the biggest changes illness or injury can cause is the inability to work. This change is difficult to adjust to because work can provide an environment for personal accomplishment, social interaction, goal structure and income. Despite these facts, people often tell them they are lucky they do not have to work.

Does it make any sense for us to say this when someone did not willingly quit their job? For most people, the loss of personal satisfaction and enjoyment of their careers can be devastating. Besides, they are faced with a loss of income and must also contend with mounting medical bills. No, it is not because someone does not *have* to work, it is because they *cannot* work.

What's more, what most people do not realize is that the brain is often affected by illness, injury or medications, as well. Many times we will say, "At least your mind is intact" or "At least your brain is not affected." Quite the opposite is true, as many have lost various degrees of cognitive abilities. Such things as memory, comprehension and word recall can be a frustrating struggle. These occurrences are commonly referred to as "brain fog:" it might feel as if cement has solidified in the brain, keeping it from operating.

In all, many people living with debilitating symptoms wrestle with the activities most people take for granted, like washing their hair, preparing themselves a meal, running an errand or going to a doctor's appointment. Let's face it. Nobody likes to be so sick or in pain that they are unable to work, shop, cook, clean or go to an activity, even if it is only for a couple of days. In view of that, let us be sensitive to people who are sick or in pain for weeks, months or even years at a time.

Do Not Disregard Their Limitations

"Come on! You can do it!" "You always say 'No'!"
"Aren't you better off when you push yourself?"
"You're just giving up!" "You need to get out more!"

When we break a leg, are we better off hopping on it or using crutches? Right after having major surgery, would we recover better if we went hiking or if we rested a bit in the hospital? We all know the answer to those questions. Otherwise, there would be mountain slopes, instead of gurneys, outside of every operating room.

However, usually when dealing with a broken leg, it heals and the person returns to life as usual. On the other hand, for many living with ongoing illness, "As the illness progresses, she must adjust each day to the disease, sometimes severe, sometimes in remission, and always present. The sense of health and vibrancy is, at best, diminished, and at worst, lost,"[19] wrote Jackson P. Rainer, a leading authority on grief and loss.

Although we might think our loved one is lazy and sleeps all day, they often have difficulty sleeping and can become sleep deprived. Thus, we need to allow them to rest whenever possible. After all, they are busy trying to maintain their condition and often have to push themselves hard to accomplish a few simple chores. With each activity they give their effort to, another could be forfeited and a price paid. After being limited for a while, they will begin to learn how to juggle their efforts and will discover what and how much causes them to hit a wall.

Notably, we need to believe them when they say they cannot do something. Because we saw them participating in a task before, does not mean they can do it again. "Only she knows her limits and they will likely change from day to day depending on many factors. What she could do yesterday may not be possible today. Don't question that."[20] Therefore, we must respect their limitations without enforcing a guilt trip when they are already trying to do more than their bodies can handle.

Do Not Claim They Are Not Trying Hard Enough

"You could get better if you wanted to."
"You should just try harder." "You're being lazy."
"You need to be more motivated."

Often when we come across someone who says they have been sick or in pain for a long time, we might think they are either exaggerating or not doing something about it. After all, when most people get sick, they get some rest, take some medication and are soon back on their feet. So why can't our loved one do that, too?

What we usually do not realize is how much a person does to attempt to regain their health. Customarily, they have seen many doctors, had several tests, tried lots of medications and have undergone various procedures. Even so, doctors do not always have all the answers. In fact, as our modern medicine improves, chronic illness actually rises. "Excellent medical care saves lives and thereby increases the rate of chronic illness."[21]

Nevertheless, we treat them as if their situation is due to a lack of motivation or attitude. We tell them if they "would just try harder," have a "better attitude" and use "mind over matter," they would not be suffering. Chronic Fatigue Immune Dysfunction Syndrome patient, Patti Schmidt, explained, "Normally, the thought of overcoming obstacles is not abhorrent to me....But with CFIDS, I found myself with something I could not 'work' around. I couldn't pretend CFIDS wasn't there. I couldn't shed it like an old skin. I couldn't even work harder to overcome it. In fact, working harder is exactly what I *shouldn't* be doing."[22]

Consequently, we should never treat our loved one as if they have chosen to have this condition and have chosen to quit taking part in activities they enjoy and miss. This approach is incredibly misconstrued, because why would they choose to give up those things they love? Most of all, why would we tell someone debilitated by their illness, "You just don't want to work," "You just don't want to go out for dinner," or "You just don't want to play with your children" when they want those things for themselves more than we could possibly want those things for them?

The truth is, if we look a little closer, we might see that our friend or family member is fighting this illness every step of the way, with courage most of us may never experience.

Do Not Act As If You Can Relate

"I know what you mean. I'm always tired, too." "Join the club."
"Ya, I can't get anything done, either."
"Hey, I would like to have a maid, too."

We all do it. For some reason, we tend to think that showing how we can relate will confirm our compassion for a person's circumstances. However, in any situation, if we have not actually been in their shoes, we cannot declare we really know what it is like. For that reason, trying to say we know how someone feels will almost always backfire, because we do not.

For this reason, when a person is not really in the same boat, many living with chronic conditions resent comments such as, "Join the club." Eileen, a woman living with Rheumatoid Arthritis declared, "…my aunt is one of those, 'I have what you have, only I have it worse,' types. Drives me nuts. No matter what you have, she's had it, has it, her husband had it, or one of her kids, only it was much worse. I haven't seen her in a while, and not since my RA diagnosis, so I'll be interested to hear how bad her RA is!"[23]

Michele, a wife and mother with severe disc degeneration in her back, added, "My mom does this 'me too' thing as well. She was out after I had my back surgery and would make comments saying she hurt this much too and just had some chiropractic treatments and was better. I just kept thinking that if she hurt as bad as I was, how could she possibly be functioning without any pain control? At that point I could barely get to the bathroom let alone try to do anything else. For the year leading up to the surgery she did the same thing."[24]

The bottom line is that a person who is not living with a disease or injury that can be incapacitating should not try to relate their normal aches, pains and tiredness with the symptoms of their loved one's condition. For example, how can a person tell a friend or family member they know how the person feels, because they are exhausted at the end of a busy day? It is true that a healthy person may be tired, but why? Probably because they got up, took a shower, got dressed, ran their vacuum, put in a load of laundry, shopped for groceries, made some phone calls, made dinner and lots more.

On the other hand, a person with a debilitating disorder can be beyond tired before they try to get anything done, because they often wrestle with horrible fatigue, nausea, cognitive dysfunctions, dizziness, weakness, excruciating pain and more. As a result, they have to push themselves to do a few of the simple things nobody else gives a thought to - such as washing their hair, getting a meal or going to a doctor's appointment. Unlike those who are well, they often do not have the satisfaction of having several accomplishments behind them at the end of the day to account for how tired they feel.

No, people with limiting conditions are not in the "well person's club." Members in that club are able to care for their own daily needs and achieve many goals without much thought as to the physical cost. Yes, they may be tired or exhausted from running around and living their life to its fullest, but many living with chronic disorders are often sick and in pain from not much activity at all.

Do Not Give Advice All the Time

"Why don't you..." "Why can't they just..."
"Can't you take something?"

At the moment a person becomes ill, they start searching out ways to get better. They see a doctor, they take vitamins or medications and they try to recuperate. If the illness does not seem to go away, they see the doctor again and try other medications. If they are still not getting relief, they may see more doctors, have more tests done and spend more money on medical bills.

After some time has passed and they are told there is nothing else that can be done, they rarely give up. They do more research, look for people who are dealing with the same things and often try what other people are using. All in all, most people keep researching, looking and hoping, because they want their lives back to normal.

Imagine being in that position and just about every time you run into a friend, family member or a stranger, you are given advice about what to do, what to eat, how to act and what to take. Senior Editor of *Arthritis Today*, Mary Anne Dunkin described, "...everyone from lifelong friends to strangers on the street claims to know more about what's good for you than you or your doctor do."[25]

What is worse is when people share the advice as if it should be a simple remedy for the situation. In other words, when we toss out a quick fix, such as, "all you need to do is this or that," we are assuming they have not thought of such an obvious idea. For example, many living with injuries or chronic pain that has become debilitating, are asked, "Why don't you just take some aspirin?" More than likely they have thought of that and not only tried it, but have tried many substances much stronger.

As a whole, this can be overwhelming and frustrating when people act as if they can come up with a solution in a minute, when you have been trying for months or years to find one. Furthermore, it makes our loved ones feel as if we think they are either not trying to find an answer ,or worse, are plain brainless.

Sometimes sharing information or contacts that helped us or someone we know, can be beneficial, especially in the beginning. Yet, we need to listen when our loved ones tell us they have "tried that already." We should not keep insisting our solution will work because it worked for our Aunt Sally. After all, not all medications, diets and therapies work for every person. We often think modern medicine has a simple answer for everyone, but this is not always true. In fact, "Chronic illness rarely responds to a direct intervention, and by definitions, is elusive of cure."[26]

Do Not Try To Tell Them How They Feel

"You look like you are feeling well!" "You must be doing better!"
"You are here, so you must be doing well!"
"You must be having a good day!"

When we try to prompt our loved one for a certain answer, we are not really asking them how they are, but telling them what we want to hear. We do this when we only want to hear they are doing well. It is easy to do, because when we see our loved one out of the house and smiling, we often assume they are having a good day.

"Of course, [people] really do believe that you must be feeling better or you wouldn't be out of bed. Those of us, who are ill, however, understand that if we stayed in bed until we felt better, we would never leave the bedroom and we would miss out on life. So we get out of bed."[27]

Instead, we must understand they cannot always wait for a "good day" to get out, because they need to get their groceries or run errands just like everyone else. We should recognize what a great effort it takes for them to get out and about, when they are feeling so badly.

"Usually people find a way to cope with sickness, not because they want to but because, if it is neither curable nor lethal, what other choice do they have?"[28] In light of that, instead of assuming when we see them that it means they are doing great, we should be aware that most likely they will probably be worse from the exertion.

For these reasons, pressuring our friend or family member to report they are doing well, despite the truth, can put them into a precarious position. They will be faced with having to choose to either lie about how they are doing or tell the truth and risk being treated as if they are being negative. Believe it or not, it is more difficult for them to live the truth, then for us to simply hear it.

Do Not Point Out What They Still Have

"At least you have..." "At least you can..."
"At least you're not..." "Look at the bright side!"
"Count your blessings!"

Many bereavement experts say that only the person grieving is allowed to start a sentence with "At least..." We agree! This proclamation must come from them and not from us. When we declare "At least..." we are ignoring and minimizing what another person is trying to express to us. Once again, these comments only cause our loved one to realize that we are unwilling to address and deal with what they are going through. When we allow them to be honest about their feelings and hear their concerns, they will trust that we comprehend their losses and situation. Only then, will they feel safe to start saying "At least I can..." or "At least I have..." on their own.

What's more, we cannot assume a person living with a continuing condition does not look at the bright side or count their blessings. As a matter of fact, people with continuing illness and pain often count blessings not thought of by most other people. For instance, do you give thanks for being able to do one load of laundry? Most people complain about having to do laundry at all and would be frustrated if they were only able to do one load once in a while. What about when you finally dusted off a couple of pieces of furniture, after weeks of it needing to be dusted? How about when you drove yourself to a doctor's appointment? Nobody likes to spend time going to a doctor's appointment: yet were you thankful you were able to drive there and back? Even more, do you count your blessings because you took a shower and made dinner all in one day? Now consider doing both tasks, knowing it will result in horrible pain, aching all over and feeling like you are going to pass out.

We must not treat our loved ones as if they have not been thankful for everything they "at least have." Instead, we should look to see their incredible will to keep going, despite all they have been through. For goodness sake, they are grateful for things that most people take for granted every single day!

Do Not Expect Them To Always Be Happy

"Just be positive!" "Don't cry!" "Cheer up!"
"Oh, you're doing fine!"

When we see our friend or family member struggling and overwhelmed with their circumstances, we often want to tell them they need to be positive. We do this because we assume their symptoms result from the lack of a good mental attitude. On the contrary, we must learn that most often their "Symptoms may be a result of fatigue more than psychological weakness."[29]

We might even criticize their sense of humor regarding their condition, as well as incidents with doctors, insurance companies and people around them. Psychiatrist Dr. Jeffrey Boyd described, "The humor I've found among sick people is difficult to reproduce. It is often a dark humor, sarcasm, irony, almost a gallows humor. Outsiders sometimes think these remarks are 'sick,' not funny."[30] Yet, Dr. Boyd lists this humor as one of his top coping strategies.

At any rate, most people cannot bear feeling sick or in pain, seeing doctors, taking medications, missing work and being unable to care for the home for more than a few days. Imagine the perseverance it takes to keep going and keep fighting when sickness and pain can last for weeks, months or years at a time. Therefore, when we tell our loved one they need a positive attitude, it can cause them to realize we have no idea what courage it has taken thus far to cope and what strength they continue to display.

Clearly, if they are not always perky or elated about their situation, please understand this is to be expected. "One of the greatest human challenges is found in the demands of an illness that becomes ruthlessly ongoing and chronic. A chronic illness accompanies every move the individual makes. It casts a constant pall over thoughts and actions."[31]

Yes, the chronically ill or injured should be able to laugh and get some enjoyment out of life and that is what they strive to do every single day. Even so, sometimes they need to stop and mourn what they have lost and properly work through their changes. "It is no wonder that many people facing these multiple losses and the grief that naturally ensues find themselves experiencing high levels of anger, fear, helplessness, hopelessness, resentment, depression and damaged self-esteem."[32]

They are living in bodies that will not always allow them to do what most can do without a thought. Many have lost friends, hobbies and even careers. Some have had to forgo life's simple privileges like dusting furniture, making meals, going shopping or showering regularly. So, let's try to be more understanding.

What Encourages Them?

Now that we have seen what kinds of comments can discourage our loved one, we are sure you are eager to find out what you can say to be an encouragement! The following is a list of guidelines to follow, what to say and why:

Acknowledge Their Situation

"What you have been through is horrible!"
"I can't believe what you contend with!"
"Yes, that must be really difficult!"

As we discussed earlier, oftentimes when a person continues to be sick or in pain for a long period of time, the people around them fail to move out of denial about the situation. Instead of acknowledging what they have been through and what they are facing on a daily basis, we refuse to hear the facts and we minimize the severity of the condition. We do this in an attempt to protect ourselves and the person suffering. Unfortunately, by doing this we are treating the person as if they are exaggerating or not being honest, when they are simply communicating what they are going through.

Sometimes we question if the disorder exists or is really as bad as the person claims. Why would we disbelieve them? When a friend says they have broken their leg, do we refuse to believe it is broken and then claim they are making it up? Probably not. Nevertheless, why is an invisible illness or injury any different? Is it because we can actually see the cast, which confirms their claim? Why do we have to have visual proof that our friend or family member is telling the truth? Don't they deserve more respect and trust than that?

If we take a look at four accompanying conditions, we can be sure our loved one is being forthright. 1) Were they an active person before the condition? 2) Do they convey their desire to be able to do those activities again? 3) Do they express their frustration with their limitations? 4) Are they actively treating their condition? If these things are true for them, then why would they suddenly go from being motivated and on-the-go to unable to do the activities they love to do?

As a whole, we must believe our loved one and acknowledge their situation, because "Facing facts, however frightening, is vital to mutual coping. You can't begin to solve a problem if one or both of you refuse to acknowledge it."[33] When we take these steps, we are addressing the facts, so we can move on to practical help. After all, no one can stand alongside a soldier to plan and execute a battle if they refuse to believe the adversary exists!

Acknowledge Their Losses

"I am so sorry you can't work anymore!"
"It must be horrible, because you can no longer..."
"I can't imagine what you have been through!"

When we do not acknowledge their losses and we remain in denial, our loved one is unable to move on to making proper adjustments. Dr. Pauline Boss cautioned, "Coping is blocked; behavioral adaptations become non-existent or dysfunctional as the family waits and wishes for a miracle to put things right again."[34]

Let's think about it. Wouldn't losing the ability to participate in activities, work or enjoy hobbies be devastating to anyone? Writer Susan Dion, who lives with CFIDS declared, "The losses go far beyond the former healthy body; they often include loss of employment, loss of income, loss of intellectual acuity, loss of former expectations, loss of social life, and so on."[35] It includes fearing more losses in the future.[36]

What people often do not realize is that those disabled by illness and pain often mourn the loss of part or much of their identity. Dion added, "Indeed, the illness results in the loss of varied parts of the self."[37] This type of loss often affects those around them as well, because the person cannot fill the shoes of their customary role in friendships and family.

Deidra expressed, "Having RSD has been a nightmare for me but I feel it has been harder on my family. I was one of those moms that worked full-time but did everything with my kids and still found time to fall in love everyday with my husband. I now consider a good day to be when I get out of bed and spend any amount of time with my family. I miss ME! I miss my relationships with my kids and especially with my husband. I always need help with everything, whereas before, I was the helper."[38]

Consequently, when we acknowledge our friend or family member's losses, we show them we recognize what they can no longer do or enjoy. It demonstrates that we believe their loss is extremely difficult to deal with and not something they have willfully chosen for themselves. Accordingly, when we address the situation and recognize it as a validated loss, "...families will be better able to construct a new meaning of their situation and move on with their lives..."[39] Boss added.

Respect Their Boundaries and Limitations

"We would like to get together, so what kinds of things do you enjoy doing?" "If you can't make it, we will understand."

Having unwanted limitations is discouraging, to say the least. The last thing anyone wants is to lose parts of their lives that make them happy and bring them joy. Even so, when a person experiences recurrent limitations, they must learn to set boundaries. "Chronic medical illness demands continuous coping and a flexible range of responses, from minimal life change to severe disruption of daily activities; even a complete life change in the presence of a chronic illness is not unusual."[40]

With time, they will discover that the price of failing to stay within those boundaries will most likely cause them to worsen and to have to give up more activities later on. Suitably, it is advised to "Find your limits. Living inside the Energy Envelope offers an alternative to the cycle of push and crash."[41] For that reason, we should not push them to do things they should not be doing, but instead respect their boundaries. Copen requested, "Respect her limitations and be sensitive to them. Don't say, 'A little walk might do you some good' or 'No pain, no gain!'"[42]

As a result, we must also remember that if a person has to say "No" to an activity, that it does not mean they do not want to participate. If they say they can't, they mean they can't. It does not mean they don't want to join in the activity. "Living with a chronic illness means that we will have to make choices to do something or to not do something every day."[43]

In fact, they despise having to say "No" to something they want to do. It tears them up inside when they have to miss out on yet another activity they would enjoy. To make matters worse, when we dispute their inability to participate, they also then have to contend with our perception that they are choosing not to go and are using the illness as an excuse.

In addition, they may have some better days than others, so we should not question how they can do something one day, but not on another day. "Chronic illness is erratic and unpredictable and requires constant readjusting."[44] They may push themselves to participate once in a great while, but that does not mean they can do that all of the time.

Does this mean we should not ask our friend or family member to go places with us because they usually say "No"; we sure hope not! If our invitations cease, they will be even more isolated, as well as feeling left out and forgotten. Of course, if they tell us they are no longer able to do a certain thing, let us not keep asking them to do it. Otherwise, as long as we are willing to accept hearing "No" either once in a while or most of the time, we need to keep asking.

Show Them You Are Aware Of Their Circumstances

"I am so glad you are here, I know it is a huge sacrifice for you!" "Wow! Thank you for coming! I know it is very difficult for you!"

When a person debilitated by their illness shows up to a gathering, you can bet they had to sacrifice a lot to get there. Unfortunately, we often meet them with comments such as, "Wow, you must be feeling better!" or "You must be having a good day!" Many times, this could not be further from the truth. They may not have the luxury of waiting until they feel good in order to get out, because that might mean they never leave the house. So, these types of comments can make them realize we are unaware of what they had to go through to get there.

In fact, the effort to make it to a gathering or to have company, and sitting, smiling and talking can be like climbing Mt. Everest. We must realize it may not be because our loved one is feeling well that they are there; it is because they desire the companionship so much that they are willing to pay the price.

Thus, when we recognize how much effort went into getting there, we are making it apparent that we are aware of the hurdles they leaped and the cost for their efforts. By doing this, they will know we appreciate their endeavor, respect their challenges and are honored by their sacrifice. We might drop them a note that confirms our enjoyment of their company. This way, when they are at home paying the price, they are reminded that it was worth it!

Show Them You Are Listening

"Honestly, how are you doing?" "How can I pray for you?"
"So, what is really going on?"

Certainly, when we see someone with a chronic condition in passing, he or she would not expect us to stand there and listen to all of their problems. On the other hand, when the time is right, we should take a moment to do so once in a while. We do not have to worry about doing this every time we talk to them or see them. In fact, they will appreciate it if we do not make it a regular part of conversation. Spending time with them is often enough. They do not always want to talk about their health issues.

We should note that it can be quite tiresome for them to continually be asked how they feel. This is especially true for those who tell us they are ill or in pain every day. We want to show our concern, but we don't know what to say. If we ask them how they are doing, this can spark an answer that addresses how they are dealing with their challenges and emotional state. This gives the person a chance to answer they are *doing well,* where as they could not if the question was about how they *feel.*

Either way, if they are not feeling well nor doing well, let's show them we care by accepting their answer, as difficult as it might be for us to hear. If we refuse to listen, it will only make their losses seem greater because now they have lost us, as well.

Yet, when we are there for them, our compassionate care is invaluable to their ability to not only cope, but to thrive. "People are happier when they have family and friends supporting them than when they feel isolated."[45] Our willingness to stand by their side to hear their concerns and not ignore them can help them gain the strength to continue the fight.

Give Them A Compliment

"You look very nice today." "I like your hair that way."
"I wish you could feel as good as you look!"

How do we give a person a compliment when it seems like every time we try, they respond with a glare as if we said something awful? As addressed previously in this booklet, we often make the mistake of connecting how a person is looking with how they are feeling. For example, when they tell us how they are feeling, we indicate doubt in what they are saying by rebutting, "But you LOOK good!"

Another time a well-intentioned compliment might be misconstrued is when we look at them and say, "You look like you are feeling great today!" That would be wonderful if it were true, but it is making an assumption that because they look good, they feel good. These comments prove we are unaware of their pain on the inside, even though they may look fine on the outside.

However, we should not give up on showering them with a flattering remark as we do for anyone else! After all, they want to look their best when they see us. They often work hard to hide their fatigue and pain under make up, combed hair, clean clothes and a smile. Therefore, let us not make the issue confusing. If we want to know how they are feeling, we should simply ask, "How are you feeling?" Conversely, if we want to tell them they look nice, we might say, "Wow, you look nice!" We can convey our understanding by adding, "I wish you could *feel* as good as you look." It is that easy. Everyone likes a good compliment now and then. So, let's give it a try.

Show Them Your Admiration

"I can't believe how strong you are!" "I can't believe how hard you keep fighting!" "You are so courageous!" "You amaze me!"

Believe it or not, it is all too common for a person living with a continuing illness or pain to be treated as if they are not positive enough, do not try hard enough, do not want to get better and do not have anything to complain about. Then again, most people cannot imagine how difficult it is to be inside a body that will not cooperate with their desires.

If we would take a moment to realize how much our loved one has been through, what they go through daily, how many tests they have had, how many doctors they have seen, how many medications they have tried, how much research they have done and how much money they have spent to battle the symptoms, we would recognize our loved one's amazing courage.

In any case, don't most people become crabby and whiney when they get sick, even though they know they will be better in a few days? Imagine having symptoms much or all of the time. Let's face it, "...an ambiguous loss of long duration becomes physically and psychologically exhausting for even the strongest of individuals, couples and families."[46] Think of how amazing this person is for having such persistence to find a way to remove or at least alleviate their symptoms and to find ways to cope. Consequently, isn't it time to voice our admiration for their incredible strength and determination? We think so!

Show Them You Are Willing To Help

"I'm going to the store, can I pick something up for you?"
"Can I bring you lunch tomorrow? Maybe you will let me wash some dishes for you while I am there!"

There are basically three reasons why we are unwilling to assist a person debilitated on an ongoing basis. First, we think they do not require assistance because they look okay, which must mean they are getting along fine. Second, we fear that helping them will require a big commitment and be too time-consuming. Third, we think it is too hard to get involved emotionally.

First of all, by reading this booklet we have already learned not to correlate how someone looks with how they feel. Next, later in the book we will learn more about how it only takes a little bit of our effort to make a big difference. Lastly, as we learn how to listen and what to say, the relationship can still be quite enjoyable.

Overall, when our loved ones struggle to undertake the tasks of a few daily needs, they often have to forgo many other necessities and enjoyable activities. Appropriately, the family and friend support system can divide their usual responsibilities and chores amongst each other. In other words, "…the healthy family member with more resilience and leeway must take the lead in adapting to fluctuating absence and presence, a situation that may not go away."[47] Read on to discover some practical ways to help.

Let Them Know You Appreciate Your Health

"You have made me realize how much I take for granted."
"You really make me appreciate being able to do things
I never even thought about before."

Let's admit it. Almost everyone complains about working, shopping, cooking and cleaning. Trying to keep up with life is tough, because there is always so much to do. Because of this, it is not out of the ordinary for people to run down a list of what they have to do, as though it is dreadful. Yet we do not always realize these responsibilities are chores a person is able to do, and that they are tasks that a person who is debilitated wishes they could do.

People who experience physical limitations realize the everyday jobs they used to complain about are and were blessings. Most everybody has been there. Even when we had surgery or were sick for a few days we grasped how much we took for granted, because it took all we had to get out of bed, get something to eat or wash our hair. We were then immensely grateful when we were able to return to our usual routine. Nonetheless, it did not take much time at all for us to forget our thankfulness for being able to do these tasks.

For those living within these constraints on a daily or regular basis, they yearn to be able to do a small portion of what everyone else takes for granted and gripes about. They long to be able to do the things people dread, like scrubbing the toilet and dusting the furniture. Likewise, they know that if they were able to regain their health, they would look at each morning as a gift and opportunity to accomplish many goals and appreciate every one they could accomplish.

As a result, it is refreshing and consoling to our loved one when people take a moment to be thankful for what they are able to do, instead of grumbling about it. Judy, a woman who was searching out information for a relative in chronic pain, shared, "I have lived with people around me with disabilities, just about all my life. I do not take for granted for me personally being healthy."[48] Moreover, it is wonderful for a person to realize they did not have to lose their abilities, in order to learn this valuable outlook.

Show Us Your Love, And We Will Show You Our Courage

Chapter Four

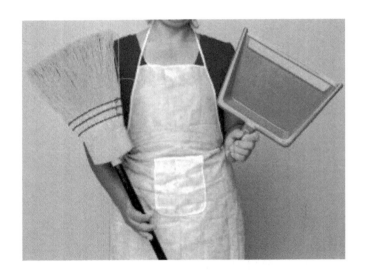

I Never Know What to Do!

You may never know what results

come of your actions,

but if you do nothing,

there will be no results.

~ Mahatma Gandhi

The Balancing Act

When a person has a long-term condition, they may lose various degrees of their ability to complete daily tasks. Some have good and bad days and may need occasional help on those bad days. Others have few good days and find it unattainable to keep up with the bare necessities.

Often when we think of someone who is sick or in pain, we think they must be sitting around with nothing to do but read and watch TV. Because of this, those living with debilitating conditions often hear comments such as, "Oh, it must be nice to be on vacation!" or "I wish I had the time to just lie around all day!" Quite the opposite is true. Don't we find that when we are sick, it is stressful to not be able to get anything done? What's more, don't the chores keep piling up?

It can be quite a challenge to have to choose which two or three of our 100 daily tasks will get done. Does this sound like your life? Think again. Try counting all of the tasks you accomplish in a day, including making your bed, hanging up clothes, putting away shoes, filing a stack of papers, taking a shower, combing your hair, getting dressed, cooking a meal, washing dishes, running the vacuum, dusting furniture, doing laundry, making phone calls, sending a birthday card, paying bills, etc. Not only can most people do all that, they are also shopping for groceries, running errands, driving the kids around and having lunch with a friend. When a person is debilitated by their condition, two tasks on the list can be an all-day endeavor.

Our loved one often struggles to get a few chores done in

addition to taking a shower, taking their medication, doing their therapies and getting themselves something to eat. Many of them spend hour after hour scheduling doctor appointments, seeing doctors, having tests done, refilling prescriptions, straightening out insurance issues and more. Adding additional chores around the house and necessary errands can become overwhelming or impossible.

Unlike most people who accomplish dozens of tasks in a day and leave few undone, our friend or family member may only be able to take on a few tasks and leave dozens undone. "When you are losing 90% percent of everything because of an illness, it is important to sort out your priorities concerning what 10 percent is worth fighting to preserve."[49]

What's more, if they want to plan a visit with a friend or attend a social gathering, even more daily sacrifices may have to be made in order to prepare for the event. They do this by avoiding any other outings or projects around the house for several days or weeks because of the energy it takes to get ready, sit, smile and talk. What is more, the exertion may exacerbate their condition for several days or weeks. Then, of course, they may end up more behind on their daily duties.

At any rate, when a person's condition is debilitating, they feel as if life is rushing by without them. While everyone else is out accomplishing their goals and fulfilling their dreams, they are occupied with maintaining their condition. In view of that, we can help alleviate their load with a little assistance now and then.

Where Do I Start?

First, as we have learned, it is difficult to recognize there is a need by simply looking at someone with an illness or injury. On the outside, they may appear physically able to accomplish any task set before them, because their fatigue, pain and other symptoms are on the inside.

As a result, we must learn not to disregard what our loved one is telling us simply because we cannot see the damaged organs, cells, muscles, bones and nervous systems from the outside. Thus, the first thing we must do is to learn to listen, without discounting what we cannot see.

Second, we often fear that helping someone will be time-consuming. We think that to make a difference, we would have to cook all their meals, run all their errands and clean their house every week. Nonetheless, there are several ways to make a big difference, without a huge time commitment.

Third, many people are genuinely willing to help, but do not know where to begin. Because of this, we often offer by saying, "Call me if you need anything." This is a great effort to reach out - but, unfortunately it does not work. For that reason, we cannot put the ball in their court and expect them to call us. So, how can we help if they will not ask when they need it?" Simple... we call them!

What Can I Do?

Our loved one may need help with rides to doctor appointments, shopping, cooking and cleaning. Getting a few chores done can seem insurmountable. What is frustrating for them is that they can spend an entire day trying to do tasks that they used to be able to do in an hour. Then, at the end of the day, they still were unable to accomplish what most people take for granted, such as getting in the shower, getting dressed, running an errand and making a meal.

When limitations arise, the family needs to evaluate each individual's responsibilities. They can do this by making a list of the household chores and redistributing the jobs. Please note these tasks could fluctuate with the person's changing needs.

Next, friends can get involved in helping, as well. Be that as it may, our loved one knows people are overextended and do not have a lot of leisure time, so they do not want to add to it by being a burden. The secret to getting them to accept our much needed help is to do something that is convenient for us.

We can do this by calling and asking, "I am going to the grocery store. Can I pick up a few things for you while I am there?" This is an incredible way to save your friend or family member days' worth of energy without going too much out of your way.

Another way to approach them is to ask, "May I stop by for a short visit with you on Tuesday? Please set aside some towels I can fold or another task while I am there!" In addition, we can try, "I need to run some errands. Can I take you to a doctor's appointment while I am out?" When they know we do not have to make a special trip for them and it is virtually effortless on our part, everyone wins.

Let's not become besieged by the thought of conquering their housekeeping challenges alone. A simple way to ease their situation is to organize a group of people to chip in for monthly cleanings. Once a month does not seem like much, but it is monumental to someone with physical limitations. Another idea is to have several people give money to a cleaning fund.

Because getting out is often too arduous, we can bring them a picnic lunch, a cup of tea, flowers or a video. If they are not feeling up to the visit, we can drop it off. We can also try doubling our dinner recipe and taking them the extras once in a while for a special treat.

Sometimes having company can be quite stressful for our loved one, because they are probably way behind in household duties. This is quite humiliating to them, because if they had any other choice, everything would be neat and clean. We can express that we truly realize they are unable to keep things the way they desire. This may help them not to feel so embarrassed.

Something most people do not think about is that many people living with chronic illness are sensitive to chemicals and toxins. When we plan to visit our friend, unless they smoke, we should not wear clothes that have smoke residue in them. We should also ask if they have any allergic, asthmatic or other reactions to perfume, cologne, cleaning products, laundry detergent, deodorant, hair spray, lotion, candles, air fresheners, etc. While we know these things might cause our nose to itch, it may make our loved one ill with severe headaches, nausea, dizziness and incredible fatigue that could last for several days.

Reading material seems like a good thing to share, but often brain-fog from an illness, pain or medications causes reading to be quite a task. We should ask if they would enjoy a book. Some people are still able to enjoy the pleasure of reading. Others cannot read most of the time, so when their minds are clearer they must use that time to catch up on other duties. On the other hand, if we took a moment to help them with some of their strenuous tasks, they would get enormous pleasure out of using that saved energy to do those things they have dearly missed... like reading a good book.

As a whole, we must remember to listen, believe what we hear, allow them to say "No" and offer specific help that is convenient for us. Do not worry about making time for hours of strenuous help. What is simple for most people could save days of excruciating work for them!

A Little Bit of Your Time,
Can Make a Big Difference to Them!

Chapter Five

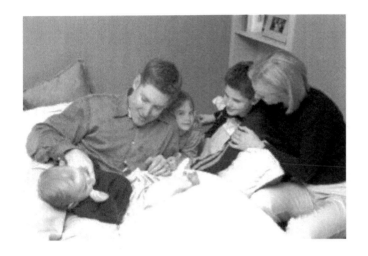

Conclusion

When in doubt ... Love

~ Peter Strople

Being a Comfort in the Storm

In all, we honestly mean well and truly want to be an encouragement and comfort to others. However, we cannot bear to see our loved one suffer. Apparently, we desperately try to believe it is not that bad and we attempt to come up with the answers to fix the problem.

We need to remember that our loved one did not choose to give up the activities they used to enjoy. In fact, they would do anything to be able to do those activities again. We can rest assured, knowing they will keep researching and pursuing ways to regain their health or at least prevent further progression of the disease.

They do not have this condition because they are weak, negative or unmotivated. Therefore, we should not claim they are sick, because they are not trying hard enough or do not have the right attitude. On the contrary, they should be commended for their perseverance to make their lives better.

We hope this booklet communicates that our natural responses, such as denial, used to protect both our loved one and ourselves, must be developed into loving acknowledgement and validation. Yes, acknowledging what is happening to our loved one may mean having to face its pain, mourning and changes. But we should not sell ourselves short. After all, if they must live with it, we can certainly live next to it!

In order for our friend or family member to learn how to cope, adjust and thrive, they must be able to assess and discuss what they are up against. In a manner of speaking, it is absolutely impossible to prepare for a climbing expedition if we keep denying the mountain even exists. Instead, we must measure the peaks and calculate the probable conditions so we can make a plan and bring the proper equipment in order to endure the journey.

Finally, once we acknowledge our loved one's situation, validate their losses, believe their word and express our desire to gain an understanding, we should see a huge change in their attitude toward both the illness and toward us. As they receive our declaration of support, our loved one can embrace our compassion and gain strength from our faith in them. Assuredly, when we stand by their side and not combatively in front of them, their fortitude can rise like a mighty warrior empowered to do battle against the relentless enemy.

NOTES:

[1] U.S. Department of Commerce: BUREAU OF THE CENSUS, "Disabilities Affect One-Fifth of All Americans: Proportions Could Increase in Coming Decades," *CENSUS BRIEF, Publication CENBR/97-5* (December 1997): 1. Found at: www.census.gov/prod/3/97pubs/cenbr975.pdf (accessed April 17, 2006). Body

[2] John M. McNeil, "Americans with Disabilities: 1994-95," Current Population Report: CENSUS BUREAU, Publication P70-61 (April 1997): 1. Found at: www.census.gov/prod/3/97pubs/p70-61.pdf (accessed April 17, 2006). Body.

[3] Rochelle Ratner, "A Private Write," *InsideMS,* (October-December 2002): 35.

[4] Fred Friendly Seminars, Inc, "What Is Chronic Illness?" *Who Cares: Chronic Illness in America* (2001). Found at , www.pbs.org/inthebalance/archives/whocares/awareness/what_is.html (accessed April 24, 2006).

[5] Ward BW, Schiller JS, Goodman RA. Multiple chronic conditions among US adults: a 2012 update. Prev Chronic Dis. 2014;11:130389. DOI: http://dx.doi.org/10.5888/pcd11.130389.

[6] Pauline Boss, "Ambiguous Loss from Chronic Physical Illness: Clinical Intervention with Couples, Individuals, and Families," *Journal of Clinical Psychology-In Session, Volume 58* (November 2002): 1352.

[7] Lynn, Personal Communication: Email to IDA (April 19, 2006), Quoted with permission granted April 21, 2006.

[8] Geri Fosseen, "Looking Good, Feeling Bad." *Melissa Kaplan's Chronic Neuroimmune Diseases.* Found at: www.anapsid.org/cnd/coping/lookgood.html (accessed March 30, 2006). Introduction.

[9] Lisa Copen, "When Friends Just Don't Understand," *...And He Will Give You Rest Newsletter,* Volume 1, Issue 4. Found at: www.restministries.org/articles/art-whenfriendsdontunderstand.htm (accessed March 3, 2006). Body.

[10] Lisa Copen, "When the Illness is Invisible," *...And He Will Give You Rest   Newsletter,* Volume II, Issue 3 (1998): www.restministries.org/art-invisible.htm (accessed March 23, 2004). Body.

[11] F. Marcus Brown, III, "Inside Every Chronic Patient Is an Acute Patient Wondering What Happened," *Journal of Clinical Psychology-In Session, Volume 58* (November 2002): 1446.

[12] Jeffrey Boyd, *Being Sick Well* (Grand Rapids, Michigan: Baker Books, 2005), 26.

[13] Karen J. Zielinski, "The Devil of Denial," *InsideMS,* Vol. 18, No. 2 (Spring 2000): 61.

[14] Copen, "When the Illness is Invisible," Introduction.

[15] Kristine, IDA Guestbook (March 2006). Quoted with permission granted 4/20/2006. Link to guestbook found at www.MyIDA.org.

[16] Fosseen, Introduction.

[17] Elaine Zablocki, "Looking Good, Feeling Rotten," *WebMD Medical News* (November 19, 2001). Found at: www.webmd.com/content/article/12/1689_51679. Introduction.

[18] Zanda Hilger, "Loss Related to Chronic Illness," *Loss and Grief Module 13.* Found at:www.familycaregiversonline.com/family_caregiver_modules.htm (accessed March 30, 2006).

[19] Jackson Rainer, "Bent but Not Broken: An Introduction to the Issue on Chronic Illness," *Journal of Clinical Psychology- In Session, Volume 58* (November 2002): 1348.

[20] Lisa Copen, "When a Friend Has a Chronic Illness," brochure by Rest Ministries, Inc. 2001. Found at: www.restministries.org/art-whattosay.htm (accessed April 22, 2006). Body.

[21] Boyd, 22.

[22] Patti Schmidt, "Coming to Terms with a Life I Didn't Plan," *CFIDS & Fibromyalgia Self Help.* Found at: http://www.cfidsselfhelp.org/artcl_success_patti.htm (accessed March 30, 2006). Introduction.

[23] Eileen, IDA's Online Support Group (March 2006). Quoted with permission granted April 13, 2006. Link to support group found at: www.MyIDA.org. Members only.

[24] Michele, IDA's Online Support Group (April 2006). Quoted with permission granted April 18, 2006. Link to support group found at: www.MyIDA.org. Members only.

[25] Mary Anne Dunkin, "The Advice Givers," *Arthritis Today,* (November-December 1999). Found at: www.arthritisfoundation.org/resources/arthritistoday/1999_archives/ 1999_11_12advice_givers.asp (accessed March 30, 2006). Introduction.

[26] Brown, 1444.

[27] Copen. "When the Illness is Invisible," Introduction.

[28] Boyd, 10.
[29] Boss, 1353.

[30] Boyd, 12.
[31] Rainer, 1347.

[32] Hilger, "Loss Related to Chronic Illness," Body.

[33] Melissa Bienvenu "Happily Ever After," *Arthritis Today* (September-October 1997).The Arthritis Foundation. Found at: www.arthritis.org/resources/happily_ever_after.asp (accessed March 30, 2006). Body.

[34] Boss, 1358.

[35] Susan Dion, "Rethinking Usefulness." *The National Link,* (Winter 1995): 1.

[36] Hilger, "Loss Related to Chronic Illness," Body.

[37] Dion, 1.

[38] Deidra, Personal Communication: Email to IDA (January 5, 2006). Quoted with permission granted on 4/22/06.

[39] Boss, 1358.

[40] Brown, 1443.

[41] CFIDS & Fibromyalgia Self Help. "Ten Keys to Coping and Recovery." Found at: www.cfidsselfhelp.org/archive_ten_keys.htm (accessed on March 30, 2006). Body.

[42] Copen, "When a Friend Has a Chronic Illness," Body.

[43] Lisa Copen, "Learning to Set Boundaries," ...And He Will Give You Rest Newsletter, Volume 5, Issue 1. Found at: www.restministries.org/articles/art-learningtoset.htm (accessed March 30, 2006). Body.

[44] Hilger, "Loss Related to Chronic Illness," Body.

[45] Boyd, 11.
[46] Boss, 1353.

[47] Boss, 1359.

[48] Judy, IDA's Online Support Group (April 2006). Quoted with permission granted April 20, 2006. Link to support group found at: www.MyIDA.org. Members only.

[49] Boyd, 11.

Made in the USA
San Bernardino, CA
05 February 2017